SCARSDALE DIET

Rapid Weight Loss Program
with Meal Plans & Recipes

James G. Moore

CONTENTS

PREFACE

In a world where countless diets promise quick results and lasting transformations, it can be overwhelming to navigate the sea of options. If you are looking for a well-established and effective diet plan that has stood the test of time, you have come to the right place.

The Scarsdale Diet has been around for decades, and its popularity has endured for a good reason—it works. This book serves as a comprehensive guide to understanding and implementing the principles of the Scarsdale Diet, providing you with the tools and knowledge to embark on a journey towards improved health and weight management.

The Scarsdale Diet is not just a temporary solution but a lifestyle change. It focuses on a balanced approach to nutrition, incorporating a variety of wholesome foods while emphasizing portion control and mindful eating. By following the guidelines outlined in this book, you can achieve weight loss, improve your overall well-being, and develop healthy habits that will last a lifetime.

Throughout the pages of this book, you will find a detailed overview of the Scarsdale Diet, including its origins, core principles, and the science behind its effectiveness. You will also discover a wide range of delicious and nutritious recipes, carefully crafted to help you make the most of your dietary journey.

I have compiled this book based on extensive research, expert insights, and personal experiences. However, it is essential to remember that each person's body and health circumstances are unique. What works for one individual may not work for another. Therefore, I encourage you to listen to your body, adapt the dietary recommendations to fit your specific needs, and seek personalized guidance from healthcare professionals.

As you embark on your Scarsdale Diet journey, remember that sustainable change takes time and commitment. Stay motivated, be patient with yourself, and embrace this opportunity to transform your relationship with food and your body.

I hope that this book will serve as a valuable resource, providing you with the information, inspiration, and practical tools you need to embark on your Scarsdale Diet journey with confidence. May it empower you to make informed choices, guide you towards healthier eating habits, and ultimately contribute to your overall well-being.

Wishing you success and happiness on your Scarsdale Diet journey!

INTRODUCTION

Overview Of The Scarsdale Diet

The Scarsdale Diet is a popular weight-loss program that gained significant attention in the 1970s. Created by Dr. Herman Tarnower, a cardiologist, the diet gained prominence due to its promise of rapid weight loss. It is a low-calorie, high-protein diet that aims to help individuals shed excess pounds quickly. The Scarsdale Diet is often classified as a fad diet due to its restrictive nature and short duration.

Purpose And Goals Of The Diet

The primary purpose of the Scarsdale Diet is to facilitate rapid weight loss. It is designed to help individuals lose up to 20 pounds (9 kilograms) within a two-week period. The diet is often used as a kick-start for individuals seeking immediate results or as a way to jumpstart a longer-term weight loss journey.

The main goal of the Scarsdale Diet is to achieve quick weight loss by restricting calorie intake, controlling portion sizes, and emphasizing high-protein foods. By following the diet's guidelines, individuals aim to create a calorie deficit, resulting in fat burning and subsequent weight reduction.

Key Principles And Concepts

1. **High Protein and Low Carbohydrate Intake:** The Scarsdale Diet places a strong emphasis on consuming high amounts of protein while limiting carbohydrates. Protein is known to promote satiety and help preserve muscle mass during weight loss. The diet encourages lean protein sources such as poultry, fish, and low-fat dairy products.

2. **Strict Calorie Restriction:** The Scarsdale Diet is characterized by a low-calorie intake, typically ranging from 800 to 1,000 calories per day. This caloric deficit is intended to induce rapid weight loss. The diet plan provides specific meal suggestions to ensure individuals stay within the prescribed calorie range.

3. **Limited Fat and Sugar Consumption:** The diet restricts the consumption of fats, especially saturated and trans fats, to promote weight loss and heart health. Additionally, it encourages individuals to minimize their sugar intake to further reduce overall calorie consumption.

4. **Portion Control and Meal Structure:** The Scarsdale Diet emphasizes portion control and structured meal planning. It provides a specific meal plan for each day, consisting of a protein source, vegetables, and a small amount of fruit. The diet restricts snacking between meals to avoid excessive calorie intake.

5. **Elimination of Starches and Processed Foods:** The diet advises against consuming starchy foods such as bread, pasta, and rice. Processed foods, high in additives and preservatives, are also

discouraged. Instead, the diet promotes whole, unprocessed foods, such as fruits, vegetables, and lean proteins.

6. **Short Duration and Two-Week Cycle:** The Scarsdale Diet is designed to be followed for a short duration of two weeks. This cycle is then repeated if further weight loss is desired. After completing the initial two-week phase, a maintenance plan is recommended to help individuals maintain their weight loss.

While the Scarsdale Diet has gained popularity for its quick results, it is important to note that it is a highly restrictive diet and may not be suitable or sustainable for everyone. It is recommended to consult with a healthcare professional before embarking on any diet plan, especially one that involves significant calorie restriction.

CHAPTER ONE

Understanding The Science Behind The Scarsdale Diet

The Scarsdale Diet is a popular weight loss program that gained prominence in the 1970s. It was developed by Dr. Herman Tarnower, a cardiologist, with the goal of helping individuals lose weight quickly and safely. The diet's approach is characterized by its low-carbohydrate, high-protein composition, along with portion control and calorie restriction. To comprehend the science behind the Scarsdale Diet, it is essential to explore its key components and their impact on weight loss, metabolism, and insulin levels.

Explanation Of The Diet's Low-Carb, High-Protein Approach

The Scarsdale Diet primarily focuses on limiting carbohydrates while emphasizing protein intake. By reducing carbohydrate consumption, the body is encouraged to utilize stored fat as an energy source, resulting in weight loss. Carbohydrates are the body's main source of energy, and when they are restricted, the body turns to alternative fuel sources. This process, known as ketosis, prompts the body to break down fat stores and produce ketones, which can be used as an energy substitute.

The high-protein component of the Scarsdale Diet serves several purposes. Firstly, protein is essential for maintaining and building lean muscle mass. When combined with regular exercise, a high-protein diet can aid in preserving muscle tissue while losing fat. Additionally, protein has a higher thermic effect than carbohydrates or fats, meaning it requires more energy to digest. This increased energy expenditure can contribute to overall calorie burn and weight loss.

How The Diet Promotes Weight Loss And Fat Burning

The Scarsdale Diet promotes weight loss through various mechanisms. Firstly, the low-carbohydrate nature of the diet leads to a reduction in insulin levels. Insulin is a hormone that regulates blood sugar levels and promotes fat storage. By limiting carbohydrates, insulin secretion is minimized, allowing the body to access and utilize stored fat for energy. This metabolic shift aids in fat burning and weight loss.

Furthermore, the high-protein component of the Scarsdale Diet helps to increase satiety and control appetite. Protein-rich foods are more filling and satisfying compared to carbohydrates or fats, which can help reduce overall calorie intake. By keeping hunger at bay, individuals are less likely to overeat or succumb to cravings, facilitating weight loss.

The Role Of Portion Control And Calorie Restriction

Portion control and calorie restriction are integral aspects of the Scarsdale Diet. Controlling portion sizes ensures that individuals consume an appropriate amount of calories while still obtaining essential nutrients. By limiting calorie intake, the body is forced to tap into its fat stores for energy, leading to weight loss.

The Scarsdale Diet provides a specific meal plan that outlines the recommended portion sizes for each food group. This structured approach eliminates the need for counting calories or extensive meal planning, simplifying the weight loss process. By adhering to the prescribed portion sizes, individuals can effectively manage their calorie intake and maintain a consistent calorie deficit, which is crucial for sustainable weight loss.

Impact On Metabolism And Insulin Levels

The Scarsdale Diet can have a significant impact on metabolism and insulin levels. By reducing carbohydrate intake, the body's reliance on glucose as an energy source is diminished. Consequently, the body starts to utilize fat stores, leading to weight loss. This metabolic shift can also enhance insulin sensitivity, which is beneficial for individuals with insulin resistance or type 2 diabetes.

Insulin sensitivity refers to the body's ability to respond to insulin efficiently. Insulin resistance, on the other hand, occurs when the body becomes less responsive to insulin's actions, resulting in elevated blood sugar levels and increased fat storage. The low-carbohydrate approach of the Scarsdale Diet can improve insulin sensitivity, potentially aiding in blood sugar management.

The Scarsdale Diet can improve insulin sensitivity, potentially aiding in blood sugar management and weight loss. By reducing carbohydrate intake, the diet helps to regulate blood sugar levels, preventing spikes and crashes that can contribute to hunger and overeating. Additionally, lower insulin levels facilitate fat burning and reduce the risk of excessive fat storage.

It's important to note that while the Scarsdale Diet may have positive effects on metabolism and insulin levels, it is crucial to consult with a healthcare professional before starting any diet plan, especially if you have any underlying health conditions or specific dietary needs.

CHAPTER TWO

Health Considerations And Consulting A Healthcare Professional

When it comes to making decisions about our health, it is essential to consider various factors and consult a healthcare professional to ensure informed choices and promote overall well-being. Here are some key aspects to consider:

1. Personal Health History: Before embarking on any health-related journey or making significant changes to your lifestyle, it is crucial to reflect on your personal health history. Consider any existing medical conditions, allergies, or dietary restrictions that may impact your choices. This self-awareness will help you tailor your approach to fit your specific needs.

2. Individual Needs and Goals: Each person is unique, and what works for one individual may not work for another. Consulting a healthcare professional allows you to gain personalized insights into your health needs and set realistic goals. Whether you want to lose weight, improve your fitness level, or manage a chronic condition, a healthcare professional can provide guidance and support.

3. Nutritional Requirements: Proper nutrition is a fundamental aspect of maintaining good health. A healthcare professional can assess your nutritional needs, considering factors such as age, sex, activity level, and any specific dietary requirements. They can help you understand the importance of a balanced diet and guide you in making appropriate food choices to meet your individual nutritional needs.

4. Physical Activity Recommendations: Regular physical activity is essential for overall well-being. Consulting a healthcare professional can help you determine the right type and intensity of exercise suitable for your current fitness level and any underlying health conditions. They can provide guidance on incorporating physical activity into your routine and offer modifications if necessary.

5. Mental and Emotional Well-being: Health is not just limited to physical aspects; mental and emotional well-being also play a significant role. A healthcare professional can offer support and resources to address stress, anxiety, or any mental health concerns you may have. They can help you develop strategies to maintain a healthy mind-body connection.

6. Preventive Care: Regular check-ups and preventive care are vital for early detection and management of potential health issues. Consulting a healthcare professional allows you to stay updated on recommended screenings, vaccinations, and health monitoring. They can provide guidance on maintaining a healthy lifestyle and offer preventive interventions when necessary.

7. Medication Management: If you are currently taking any medications, it is essential to discuss them with a healthcare professional. They can provide guidance on any potential interactions with your lifestyle changes, including diet and exercise. Additionally, they can help you manage your medication schedule and monitor any side effects that may arise.

Remember, a healthcare professional is trained to provide evidence-based advice and support. By consulting them, you can make more informed decisions about your health, set realistic goals, and receive guidance tailored to your specific needs. Prioritizing your health by seeking professional input sets a strong foundation for a successful journey towards well-being.

Setting Realistic Goals And Expectations

Setting realistic goals and expectations is a crucial aspect of any endeavor, including health and lifestyle changes. Here are some key points to consider when establishing goals:

1. **Assess Your Starting Point:** Before setting goals, it is essential to assess your current situation. Evaluate your current habits, routines, and lifestyle factors that may be affecting your health. This self-reflection allows you to identify areas that require improvement and sets the foundation for establishing realistic goals.

2. **Define Specific and Measurable Goals:** Vague goals are challenging to track and achieve. Instead, set specific and measurable goals that can be objectively evaluated. For example, instead of setting a goal to "exercise more," specify a target like "walk for 30 minutes five days a week." This clarity helps you track your progress and stay motivated.

3. **Prioritize Long-term Sustainability:** While it can be

tempting to pursue rapid results, it is important to prioritize long-term sustainability in your goal setting. Consider making lifestyle changes that you can maintain in the long run rather than opting for short-term, drastic measures. This approach promotes healthier habits and ensures that your progress is sustainable over time.

4. Break It Down into Smaller Steps: Big goals can be overwhelming, and it's easy to lose motivation along the way. Break down your main goal into smaller, manageable steps. This allows you to celebrate incremental achievements and keeps you motivated as you progress. Each small step taken brings you closer to your ultimate goal.

5. Be Realistic and Flexible: It's crucial to set goals that are attainable and realistic within your current circumstances. Consider factors such as your lifestyle, time commitments, and resources available. Setting unattainable goals only sets you up for disappointment and can hinder your progress. Additionally, be flexible and open to adjusting your goals as needed to accommodate any unforeseen challenges or changes in circumstances.

6. Focus on Behavior Change: Instead of solely focusing on outcomes or numbers, shift your focus to behavior change. Sustainable results come from making lasting changes to your habits and mindset. Concentrate on developing healthier behaviors, such as incorporating more fruits and vegetables into your diet, practicing portion control, or engaging in regular physical activity. By focusing on behavior change, you lay the foundation for long-term success.

7. Celebrate Non-Scale Victories: While weight loss or specific physical measurements may be a part of your goals, don't overlook the importance of non-scale victories. Acknowledge and celebrate the positive changes you experience along the way, such as increased energy levels, improved mood, better sleep, or enhanced fitness performance. Recognizing these non-scale victories helps to keep you motivated and reinforces the positive impact of your efforts.

Setting realistic goals and expectations is essential for sustainable progress. By assessing your starting point, defining specific goals, prioritizing sustainability, breaking it down into smaller steps, being realistic and flexible, focusing on behavior change, celebrating non-scale victories, seeking support and accountability, and learning from setbacks, you create a solid framework for achieving your health and lifestyle goals.

Creating A Meal Plan And Grocery Shopping List

Creating a meal plan and a grocery shopping list are practical strategies that can support your health goals, promote balanced nutrition, and simplify your food choices. Here's how to get started:

1. Assess Your Dietary Needs and Preferences: Consider your dietary needs, including any specific dietary restrictions, allergies, or personal preferences. This assessment will help you tailor your meal plan to suit your individual requirements and ensure that you enjoy the foods you eat.

2. Set Your Meal Planning Schedule: Determine how often

you want to plan your meals. Some people prefer planning on a weekly basis, while others find it helpful to plan for the entire month. Find a schedule that works best for you and allows you to stay organized and prepared.

3. Plan Your Meals: Start by outlining your meals for each day, including breakfast, lunch, dinner, and snacks.

4. Consider Balanced Nutrition: Aim for a balanced meal plan that includes a variety of nutrients from different food groups. Include lean proteins, whole grains, fruits, vegetables, and healthy fats in your meals. Strive for a colorful and diverse plate to ensure you're getting a wide range of vitamins, minerals, and antioxidants.

5. Portion Control: Pay attention to portion sizes to maintain a healthy calorie balance. Use measuring cups, food scales, or visual cues to guide your portion sizes. Remember that portion control plays a significant role in maintaining a healthy weight and overall well-being.

6. Plan for Meal Prep: If you have a busy schedule, consider incorporating meal prep into your routine. Dedicate a specific day or time to prepare larger batches of meals or ingredients that can be used throughout the week. This practice saves time, ensures you have healthy options readily available, and reduces the likelihood of relying on convenient but less nutritious choices.

7. Variety and Flexibility: Incorporate variety in your meal plan to keep things interesting and prevent boredom. Experiment with new recipes, flavors, and cooking techniques. Additionally, allow flexibility in your plan to accommodate unexpected events or changes in your schedule. This flexibility helps you adapt and make healthier choices even in challenging situations.

8. Create a Grocery Shopping List: Once your meal plan is ready, create a grocery shopping list. Organize your list based on food categories to make the shopping experience efficient. Stick to your list to avoid impulse purchases and ensure you have all the necessary ingredients for your planned meals.

9. Shop with Nutrition in Mind: When grocery shopping, focus on nutrient-dense foods. Choose fresh produce, lean proteins, whole grains, and minimally processed foods. Read food labels to make informed choices and be mindful of added sugars, unhealthy fats, and sodium content.

Creating a meal plan and grocery shopping list sets you up for success in making healthier food choices. It promotes balanced nutrition, portion control, meal prep, variety, and flexibility. By shopping with nutrition in mind, stocking up on staples, choosing seasonal produce, and planning for healthy snacks, you ensure that your kitchen is filled with nourishing options that align with your health goals.

Tips For Successful Implementation And Adherence

Implementing and adhering to your health and lifestyle goals can be challenging, but with the right strategies, it becomes more manageable. Here are some tips to help you succeed:

1. Start with Small Changes: Begin by incorporating small, achievable changes into your routine. Gradual progress is more sustainable and helps you build momentum. For example, start by adding an extra serving of vegetables to your meals or swapping sugary drinks for water.

2. Set Reminders and Create Habits: Use reminders and cues to help you stay on track. Set alarms, use smartphone apps, or write sticky notes as visual reminders for your goals and action steps. For example, you can set a reminder to go for a walk after dinner or place a sticky note on your refrigerator as a reminder to choose healthy snacks. Over time, these reminders become habits, making it easier to stay consistent.

3. Find an Accountability Partner: Having someone to hold you accountable can greatly increase your chances of success. Share your goals and progress with a friend, family member, or join a support group. Regular check-ins and mutual support can help you stay motivated and committed to your health journey.

4. Track Your Progress: Keep a record of your progress to track your achievements and identify areas for improvement. This can be done through a journal, a mobile app, or a fitness tracker. Tracking your food intake, physical activity, and emotions can provide valuable insights and help you make necessary adjustments along the way.

5. Celebrate Milestones: Celebrate your achievements, no matter how small they may seem. Recognize and reward yourself when you reach milestones or accomplish specific goals. Celebrations can be as simple as treating yourself to a relaxing bath, buying a new workout outfit, or enjoying a healthy meal at your favorite restaurant.

6. Practice Mindful Eating: Develop a mindful eating practice by paying attention to your body's hunger and fullness cues. Slow down during meals, savor each bite, and listen to your body's signals. This practice helps prevent overeating and promotes a healthier relationship with food.

7. Find Enjoyable Activities: Engage in physical activities that you genuinely enjoy. It could be dancing, swimming, hiking, or playing a sport. When you find pleasure in the activities you choose, you're more likely to stick with them in the long run. Experiment with different activities until you find what brings you joy and keeps you motivated.

8. Manage Stress: Stress can often derail our efforts to maintain a healthy lifestyle. Find healthy coping mechanisms that work for you, such as practicing meditation, deep breathing exercises, yoga, or engaging in hobbies that help you relax. Taking care of your mental and emotional well-being is crucial for overall health and adherence to your goals.

9. Be Kind to Yourself: Remember that progress is not always linear, and setbacks are a natural part of the journey. Be kind and compassionate to yourself when faced with challenges or temporary setbacks. Instead of dwelling on mistakes, focus on learning from them and using them as opportunities for growth.

10. Seek Professional Support: If you're facing difficulties in implementing or adhering to your health goals, don't hesitate to seek professional support. A healthcare professional, registered dietitian, or a certified fitness coach can provide guidance, personalized advice, and tailored strategies to help you overcome obstacles and achieve your goals.

Implementing and adhering to your health goals requires commitment, patience, and a positive mindset. By starting small, setting reminders, finding accountability, tracking your progress, celebrating milestones, practicing mindful eating, finding enjoyable activities, managing stress, being kind to yourself, and seeking professional support when needed, you increase your chances of success and create sustainable lifestyle changes for improved health and well-being.

CHAPTER THREE

Detailed Breakdown Of The Two-Week Meal Plan

Creating a well-balanced and nutritious meal plan is essential for maintaining a healthy lifestyle. A two-week meal plan can provide structure and help individuals make healthier food choices. This article will provide a detailed breakdown of a two-week meal plan, focusing on sample menus for breakfast, lunch, and dinner for each of the seven days. By following this meal plan, individuals can ensure they are consuming a variety of nutrients and enjoying delicious meals.

Day 1

Breakfast

- Oatmeal with fresh berries, sliced almonds, and a drizzle of honey.
- A glass of freshly squeezed orange juice.

Lunch

- Grilled chicken salad with mixed greens, cherry tomatoes, cucumber slices, and balsamic vinaigrette.

- Whole-grain bread.

Dinner

- Baked salmon with lemon and herbs.
- Roasted sweet potatoes and steamed broccoli.
- A side of quinoa.

Day 2

Breakfast

- Veggie omelet with bell peppers, spinach, onions, and feta cheese.
- Whole-grain toast.

Lunch

- Quinoa and black bean burrito bowl with avocado, salsa, and a squeeze of lime.
- Mixed green salad.

Dinner

- Grilled lean steak with chimichurri sauce.
- Roasted Brussels sprouts and cauliflower.
- Brown rice.

Day 3

Breakfast

- Greek yogurt with granola, sliced banana, and a sprinkle of chia seeds.
- A cup of green tea.

Lunch

- Whole-grain wrap with turkey, hummus, spinach, and roasted red peppers.
- Carrot sticks.

Dinner

- Lentil curry with brown rice.
- Steamed asparagus.

Day 4

Breakfast

- Whole-wheat pancakes topped with fresh berries and a dollop of Greek yogurt.
- A glass of almond milk.

Lunch

- Spinach and feta stuffed chicken breast.
- Quinoa salad with diced vegetables.

Dinner

- Baked cod with a lemon and herb crust.
- Roasted butternut squash and sautéed kale.
- Couscous.

Day 5

Breakfast

- Avocado toast with sliced tomatoes and a sprinkle of sea salt.
- A cup of herbal tea.

Lunch

- Caprese salad with fresh mozzarella, tomatoes, and basil.
- Whole-grain breadsticks.

Dinner

- Grilled shrimp skewers with a garlic and herb marinade.
- Grilled zucchini and bell peppers.
- Whole-wheat couscous.

Day 6

Breakfast

- Vegetable frittata with mushrooms, spinach, bell peppers, and goat cheese.
- A glass of freshly squeezed orange juice.

Lunch

- Chickpea and vegetable stir-fry with a sesame ginger sauce.
- Brown rice.

Dinner

- Baked chicken breast with a tomato and basil sauce.
- Steamed broccoli and cauliflower.
- Quinoa.

Day 7

Breakfast

- Overnight oats with almond milk, chia seeds, and a mix of dried fruits.
- A cup of green tea.

Lunch

- Grilled vegetable wrap with hummus and feta cheese.
- Mixed green salad.

Dinner

- Baked tofu with teriyaki sauce.
- Stir-fried bok choy and snow peas.
- Brown rice.

Sample Menus And Recipes For Breakfast, Lunch, And Dinner For The Scarsdale Diet

Grilled chicken breast with steamed broccoli

Description of the meal: Grilled chicken breast with steamed broccoli is a healthy and satisfying meal that combines lean protein and nutritious vegetables. The chicken breast is marinated and grilled to perfection, resulting in a tender and flavorful main dish. The steamed broccoli provides a vibrant and crunchy side that complements the chicken perfectly.

Ingredients:

- 2 chicken breasts
- Salt and pepper to taste
- 2 tablespoons olive oil
- 1 clove garlic, minced
- 1 teaspoon dried oregano
- 1 teaspoon paprika
- 2 cups broccoli florets

Instructions:

1. Preheat the grill to medium-high heat.
2. Season the chicken breasts with salt and pepper on both sides.
3. In a small bowl, whisk together the olive oil, minced garlic, dried oregano, and paprika.
4. Brush the chicken breasts with the marinade on both sides.

5. Place the chicken breasts on the preheated grill and cook for about 6-8 minutes per side, or until the internal temperature reaches 165°F (74°C).

6. While the chicken is grilling, steam the broccoli florets until they are tender yet still crisp, about 4-5 minutes.

7. Remove the chicken from the grill and let it rest for a few minutes before slicing.

8. Serve the grilled chicken breast with steamed broccoli on the side.

Nutritional Information:

- Calories: 300
- Protein: 40g
- Fat: 10g
- Carbohydrates: 10g
- Fiber: 4g

Baked salmon with roasted asparagus

Description of the meal: Baked salmon with roasted asparagus is a flavorful and nutritious dish that is quick and easy to prepare. The salmon fillets are seasoned and baked to perfection, resulting in moist and flaky fish. The roasted asparagus adds a deliciously crisp and tender side to complete the meal.

Ingredients:

- 2 salmon fillets
- Salt and pepper to taste
- 1 tablespoon olive oil
- 1 lemon, sliced
- 1 pound asparagus spears

Instructions:

1. Preheat the oven to 400°F (200°C).

2. Season the salmon fillets with salt and pepper on both sides.

3. Drizzle the olive oil over the salmon fillets and rub it in to coat them evenly.

4. Place the salmon fillets on a baking sheet lined with parchment paper.

5. Arrange the lemon slices on top of the salmon fillets.

6. Trim the ends of the asparagus spears and place them on the baking sheet next to the salmon.

7. Drizzle the asparagus with olive oil and season with salt and pepper.

8. Bake in the preheated oven for about 12-15 minutes, or until the salmon is cooked through and flakes easily with a fork.

9. Remove from the oven and let it rest for a few minutes before serving.

Nutritional Information:

- Calories: 350
- Protein: 30g
- Fat: 20g
- Carbohydrates: 10g
- Fiber: 5g

Lean turkey meatballs with mixed greens salad

Description of the meal: Lean turkey meatballs with mixed greens salad is a light and flavorful meal that combines lean protein with a refreshing salad. The turkey meatballs are made with a blend of herbs and spices, resulting in tender and juicy bites. The mixed greens salad adds a fresh and vibrant element to the dish.

Ingredients: For the turkey meatballs:

- 1/4 cup breadcrumbs
- 1/4 cup grated Parmesan cheese
- 1/4 cup chopped fresh parsley
- 1/4 cup finely chopped onion
- 1 clove garlic, minced
- 1 teaspoon dried oregano
- 1/2 teaspoon salt
- 1/4 teaspoon black pepper
- 1 large egg, lightly beaten

For the mixed greens salad:

- 4 cups mixed salad greens
- 1 cup cherry tomatoes, halved
- 1/2 cup cucumber, sliced
- 1/4 cup red onion, thinly sliced
- 2 tablespoons extra virgin olive oil
- 1 tablespoon balsamic vinegar
- Salt and pepper to taste

Instructions

- In a large bowl, combine the ground turkey, breadcrumbs, grated Parmesan cheese, chopped parsley, chopped onion, minced garlic, dried oregano, salt, black pepper, and beaten egg. Mix until all the ingredients are well combined.
- Shape the turkey mixture into meatballs of your

desired size.

- Heat a non-stick skillet over medium heat and lightly coat it with cooking spray.
- Add the turkey meatballs to the skillet and cook for about 8-10 minutes, turning occasionally, until they are browned and cooked through.
- While the meatballs are cooking, prepare the mixed greens salad. In a large salad bowl, combine the mixed salad greens, cherry tomatoes, sliced cucumber, and thinly sliced red onion.
- In a small bowl, whisk together the extra virgin olive oil, balsamic vinegar, salt, and pepper to make the dressing.
- Drizzle the dressing over the salad and toss gently to coat.
- Serve the lean turkey meatballs alongside the mixed greens salad.

Nutritional Information:

- Calories: 350
- Protein: 25g
- Fat: 15g
- Carbohydrates: 20g
- Fiber: 5g

Instructions

- In a large bowl, combine the ground turkey, breadcrumbs, grated Parmesan cheese, chopped parsley, chopped onion, minced garlic, dried oregano, salt, black pepper, and beaten egg. Mix until all the ingredients are well combined.
- Shape the turkey mixture into meatballs of your desired size.

- Heat a non-stick skillet over medium heat and lightly coat it with cooking spray.
- Add the turkey meatballs to the skillet and cook for about 8-10 minutes, turning occasionally, until they are browned and cooked through.
- While the meatballs are cooking, prepare the mixed greens salad. In a large salad bowl, combine the mixed salad greens, cherry tomatoes, sliced cucumber, and thinly sliced red onion.
- In a small bowl, whisk together the extra virgin olive oil, balsamic vinegar, salt, and pepper to make the dressing.
- Drizzle the dressing over the salad and toss gently to coat.
- Serve the lean turkey meatballs alongside the mixed greens salad.

Nutritional Information:

- Calories: 350
- Protein: 25g
- Fat: 15g
- Carbohydrates: 20g
- Fiber: 5g

Instructions

- In a large bowl, combine the ground turkey, breadcrumbs, grated Parmesan cheese, chopped parsley, chopped onion, minced garlic, dried oregano, salt, black pepper, and beaten egg. Mix until all the ingredients are well combined.

- Shape the turkey mixture into meatballs of your desired size.

- Heat a non-stick skillet over medium heat and lightly coat it with cooking spray.

- Add the turkey meatballs to the skillet and cook for about 8-10 minutes, turning occasionally, until they are browned and cooked through.

- While the meatballs are cooking, prepare the mixed greens salad. In a large salad bowl, combine the mixed salad greens, cherry tomatoes, sliced cucumber, and thinly sliced red onion.

- In a small bowl, whisk together the extra virgin olive oil, balsamic vinegar, salt, and pepper to make the dressing.

- Drizzle the dressing over the salad and toss gently to coat.

- Serve the lean turkey meatballs alongside the mixed greens salad.

Nutritional Information:

- Calories: 350
- Protein: 25g
- Fat: 15g
- Carbohydrates: 20g
- Fiber: 5g

Grilled sirloin steak with sautéed spinach

Description of the meal: Grilled sirloin steak with sautéed spinach is a hearty and flavorful dish that combines juicy steak with nutritious greens. The sirloin steak is seasoned and grilled to perfection, resulting in a tender and flavorful main course. The sautéed spinach adds a vibrant and healthy side that pairs well with the steak.

Ingredients:

- 2 sirloin steaks
- Salt and pepper to taste
- 2 tablespoons olive oil
- 2 cloves garlic, minced
- 1 pound fresh spinach leaves

Instructions:

- Preheat the grill to medium-high heat.
- Season the sirloin steaks with salt and pepper on both sides.
- Drizzle the steaks with olive oil and rub it in to coat them evenly.
- Place the steaks on the preheated grill and cook for about 4-6 minutes per side, depending on the desired doneness.
- While the steaks are grilling, heat a large skillet over medium heat and add the minced garlic.
- Sauté the garlic for about 1 minute until fragrant.
- Add the fresh spinach leaves to the skillet and cook until wilted, stirring occasionally, for about 2-3 minutes.
- Remove the steaks from the grill and let them rest for a few minutes before slicing.
- Serve the grilled sirloin steak with sautéed spinach on the side.

Nutritional Information:

- Calories: 400
- Protein: 40g
- Fat: 20g
- Carbohydrates: 10g
- Fiber: 4g

Baked cod with lemon and dill, served with steamed green beans

Description of the meal: Baked cod with lemon and dill is a light and flavorful dish that highlights the delicate taste of the fish. The cod fillets are seasoned with fresh lemon juice and dill, then baked to perfection. Served with steamed green beans, this meal provides a healthy and satisfying combination of protein and vegetables.

Ingredients:

- 2 cod fillets
- Salt and pepper to taste
- 2 tablespoons lemon juice
- 1 tablespoon fresh dill, chopped
- 1 tablespoon olive oil
- 1 pound green beans, trimmed

Instructions:

1. Preheat the oven to 400°F (200°C).
2. Season the cod fillets with salt and pepper on both sides.
3. Place the cod fillets in a baking dish.
4. Drizzle the lemon juice over the cod fillets, then sprinkle them with fresh dill.
5. Drizzle the olive oil over the cod fillets.

6. Bake the cod in the preheated oven for about 12-15 minutes, or until it is opaque and flakes easily with a fork.

7. While the cod is baking, steam the green beans until they are tender-crisp, about 5-7 minutes.

8. Remove the cod from the oven and let it rest for a few minutes before serving.

9. Serve the baked cod with lemon and dill alongside the steamed green beans.

Nutritional Information:

- Calories: 250
- Protein: 30g
- Fat: 8g
- Carbohydrates: 10g
- Fiber: 5g

Grilled shrimp skewers with zucchini noodles

Description of the meal: Grilled shrimp skewers with zucchini noodles is a light and flavorful dish that combines succulent shrimp with a healthy alternative to pasta. The shrimp is marinated, threaded onto skewers, and grilled to perfection, while the zucchini noodles provide a refreshing and low-carb base. This dish is packed with protein and nutrients, making it a satisfying and nutritious choice.

Ingredients:

- 1 pound large shrimp, peeled and deveined
- 2 tablespoons olive oil
- 2 cloves garlic, minced
- 1 tablespoon lemon juice
- 1 teaspoon paprika

- Salt and pepper to taste
- 2-3 zucchini, spiralized into noodles
- Fresh parsley, chopped (for garnish)

Instructions:

1. Preheat the grill to medium-high heat.

2. In a bowl, combine the olive oil, minced garlic, lemon juice, paprika, salt, and pepper. Mix well.

3. Add the shrimp to the bowl and toss to coat them in the marinade. Let them marinate for about 15-20 minutes.

4. Thread the marinated shrimp onto skewers.

5. Place the shrimp skewers on the preheated grill and cook for about 2-3 minutes per side, or until they are pink and opaque.

6. While the shrimp is grilling, prepare the zucchini noodles using a spiralizer.

7. Heat a large skillet over medium heat and add a drizzle of olive oil.

8. Add the zucchini noodles to the skillet and sauté for about 3-4 minutes, until they are tender but still slightly crisp.

9. Season the zucchini noodles with salt and pepper to taste.

10. Remove the shrimp skewers from the grill.

11. Serve the grilled shrimp skewers over a bed of zucchini noodles.

12. Garnish with freshly chopped parsley.

Nutritional Information:

- Calories: 200
- Protein: 25g
- Fat: 8g
- Carbohydrates: 10g
- Fiber: 4g

Oven-roasted chicken thighs with Brussels sprouts

Description of the meal: Oven-roasted chicken thighs with Brussels sprouts is a comforting and nutritious dish that brings together tender chicken thighs with roasted Brussels sprouts. The chicken thighs are seasoned and baked to perfection, resulting in juicy and flavorful meat. The Brussels sprouts add a delicious and healthy side that complements the chicken beautifully.

Ingredients:

- 4 chicken thighs, bone-in and skin-on
- Salt and pepper to taste
- 1 teaspoon garlic powder
- 1 teaspoon smoked paprika
- 1/2 teaspoon dried thyme
- 1/2 teaspoon dried rosemary
- 1 pound Brussels sprouts, trimmed and halved
- 2 tablespoons olive oil
- 2 cloves garlic, minced

Instructions:

1. Preheat the oven to 425°F (220°C).

2. Season the chicken thighs with salt, pepper, garlic powder, smoked paprika, dried thyme, and dried rosemary. Ensure they are coated evenly.

3. In a large oven-safe skillet or baking dish, arrange the seasoned chicken thighs.

4. In a bowl, toss the Brussels sprouts with olive oil, minced garlic, salt, and pepper.

5. Arrange the Brussels sprouts around the chicken thighs in the skillet or baking dish.

6. Place the skillet or baking dish in the preheated oven and roast for about 30-35 minutes, or until the chicken is cooked through and the Brussels sprouts are tender and slightly browned.

7. Remove the dish from the oven and let it rest for a few minutes.

8. Serve the oven-roasted chicken thighs with Brussels sprouts.

Nutritional Information:

- Calories: 400
- Protein: 25g
- Fat: 25g
- Carbohydrates: 15g
- Fiber: 6g

Turkey chili with a side of mixed vegetables

Description of the meal: Turkey chili with a side of mixed vegetables is a hearty and satisfying dish that combines lean ground turkey with a flavorful blend of spices and vegetables. This chili is packed with protein and fiber, making it a nutritious choice. Served with a side of mixed vegetables, this meal provides a well-rounded balance of flavors and nutrients.

Ingredients:

- 1 tablespoon olive oil
- 1 onion, diced
- 2 cloves garlic, minced
- 1 pound lean ground turkey
- 1 can (15 ounces) kidney beans, rinsed and drained
- 1 can (15 ounces) diced tomatoes
- 1 can (6 ounces) tomato paste
- 1 cup low-sodium chicken broth
- 1 tablespoon chili powder
- 1 teaspoon ground cumin
- 1 teaspoon paprika
- Salt and pepper to taste
- Mixed vegetables of your choice (e.g., carrots, bell peppers, zucchini)

Instructions:

1. In a large pot, heat the olive oil over medium heat.

2. Add the diced onion and minced garlic to the pot. Sauté until the onion is translucent and fragrant.

3. Add the ground turkey to the pot and cook until it is browned, breaking it up with a spoon.

4. Stir in the kidney beans, diced tomatoes, tomato paste, chicken broth, chili powder, ground cumin, paprika, salt, and pepper.

5. Bring the mixture to a boil, then reduce the heat to low. Cover the pot and let the chili simmer for about 30 minutes, stirring occasionally.

6. While the chili is simmering, prepare the mixed vegetables. Wash and chop the vegetables into bite-sized pieces.

7. Steam or sauté the mixed vegetables until they are tender-crisp.

8. Season the mixed vegetables with salt and pepper to taste.

9. Serve the turkey chili alongside the mixed vegetables.

Nutritional Information:

- Calories: 350
- Protein: 30g
- Fat: 10g
- Carbohydrates: 35g
- Fiber: 10g

Baked tilapia with cauliflower rice

Description of the meal: Baked tilapia with cauliflower rice is a light and healthy dish that features tender tilapia fillets with a flavorful twist on traditional rice. The tilapia is seasoned and baked to perfection, while the cauliflower rice provides a low-carb and nutrient-rich alternative. This dish is not only delicious but also packed with protein and essential nutrients.

Ingredients:

- 4 tilapia fillets
- Salt and pepper to taste
- 1 teaspoon garlic powder

- 1 teaspoon paprika
- 1 tablespoon lemon juice
- 1 tablespoon olive oil
- 1 head cauliflower, grated or processed into rice-like texture
- 2 tablespoons butter
- 2 cloves garlic, minced
- Fresh parsley, chopped (for garnish)

Instructions:

1. Preheat the oven to 400°F (200°C).

2. Season the tilapia fillets with salt, pepper, garlic powder, and paprika on both sides.

3. Drizzle the lemon juice and olive oil over the tilapia fillets.

4. Place the seasoned tilapia fillets on a baking sheet lined with parchment paper.

5. Bake the tilapia in the preheated oven for about 12-15 minutes, or until it is opaque and flakes easily with a fork.

6. While the tilapia is baking, prepare the cauliflower rice. Grate or process the cauliflower into rice-like texture using a food processor.

7. In a large skillet, melt the butter over medium heat.

8. Add the minced garlic to the skillet and sauté for about 1 minute until fragrant.

9. Add the cauliflower rice to the skillet and cook for about 5-7 minutes, stirring occasionally, until it is tender.

10. Season the cauliflower rice with salt and pepper to taste.

11. Remove the tilapia from the oven and let it rest for a few minutes.

12. Serve the baked tilapia with cauliflower rice.

13. Garnish with freshly chopped parsley.

Nutritional Information:

- Calories: 250
- Protein: 30g
- Fat: 10g
- Carbohydrates: 10g
- Fiber: 5g

Grilled lean pork chops with steamed broccoli florets

Description of the meal: Grilled lean pork chops with steamed broccoli florets is a delicious and balanced meal that combines tender pork chops with nutritious broccoli. The pork chops are seasoned and grilled to perfection, resulting in juicy and flavorful meat. Served with steamed broccoli florets, this meal provides a satisfying blend of protein and vegetables.

Ingredients:

- 4 lean pork chops
- Salt and pepper to taste
- 2 teaspoons olive oil
- 1 teaspoon dried thyme
- 1 teaspoon paprika
- 1/2 teaspoon garlic powder

- 1/2 teaspoon onion powder
- 1 pound broccoli florets
- Lemon wedges (for serving)

Instructions:

1. Preheat the grill to medium-high heat.

2. Season the pork chops with salt, pepper, dried thyme, paprika, garlic powder, and onion powder on both sides.

3. Drizzle the olive oil over the pork chops and rub it in to coat them evenly.

4. Place the pork chops on the preheated grill and cook for about 4-5 minutes per side, or until they reach an internal temperature of 145°F (63°C).

5. While the pork chops are grilling, steam the broccoli florets until they are tender-crisp, about 5-7 minutes.

6. Season the steamed broccoli with salt and pepper to taste.

7. Remove the pork chops from the grill and let them rest for a few minutes.

8. Serve the grilled lean pork chops with steamed broccoli florets.

9. Squeeze fresh lemon juice from the lemon wedges over the pork chops for added flavor, if desired.

Nutritional Information:

- Calories: 300
- Protein: 35g
- Fat: 12g

- Carbohydrates: 10g
- Fiber: 5g

Vegetable stir-fry with tofu or chicken

Description of the meal: Vegetable stir-fry with tofu or chicken is a flavorful and nutritious dish that showcases a vibrant mix of fresh vegetables and protein. This stir-fry is a versatile recipe that allows you to choose between tofu or chicken as the protein source. The vegetables are quickly cooked in a savory sauce, resulting in a colorful and satisfying meal.

Ingredients:

- 1 block of firm tofu, cubed (or 1 pound boneless, skinless chicken breast, thinly sliced)
- 2 tablespoons soy sauce
- 1 tablespoon sesame oil
- 1 tablespoon cornstarch
- 2 tablespoons vegetable oil
- 1 onion, sliced
- 2 bell peppers, sliced
- 2 cups broccoli florets
- 1 carrot, sliced
- 2 cloves garlic, minced
- 1 tablespoon grated ginger
- 1/4 cup low-sodium chicken or vegetable broth
- 2 tablespoons oyster sauce (or soy sauce for a vegetarian version)
- 1 tablespoon honey (or maple syrup for a vegan version)
- Salt and pepper to taste

- Optional toppings: sesame seeds, chopped green onions

Instructions:

1. If using tofu, press it between paper towels to remove excess moisture. Cut the tofu into cubes.

2. In a bowl, whisk together the soy sauce, sesame oil, and cornstarch. Add the tofu cubes (or sliced chicken) to the bowl and toss to coat. Set aside.

3. Heat the vegetable oil in a large skillet or wok over medium-high heat.

4. Add the sliced onion and bell peppers to the skillet. Stir-fry for about 2-3 minutes until they begin to soften.

5. Add the broccoli florets and sliced carrot to the skillet. Continue stir-frying for another 2-3 minutes.

6. Push the vegetables to one side of the skillet and add the minced garlic and grated ginger to the cleared space. Cook for about 30 seconds until fragrant.

7. Add the tofu cubes (or sliced chicken) to the skillet, along with any remaining marinade from the bowl. Stir-fry until the tofu or chicken is cooked through.

8. In a small bowl, whisk together the chicken or vegetable broth, oyster sauce (or soy sauce), and honey (or maple syrup). Pour the sauce over the stir-fry and toss to coat the ingredients evenly.

9. Season with salt and pepper to taste.

10. Continue stir-frying for another 1-2 minutes until the sauce has thickened and the vegetables are cooked to your desired tenderness.

11. Remove the skillet from the heat.

12. Serve the vegetable stir-fry with tofu or chicken hot, garnished with sesame seeds and chopped green onions, if desired.

Nutritional Information (with tofu):

- Calories: 250
- Protein: 15g
- Fat: 12g
- Carbohydrates: 25g
- Fiber: 7g

Nutritional Information (with chicken):

- Calories: 300
- Protein: 25g
- Fat: 10g
- Carbohydrates: 25g
- Fiber: 7g

Grilled shrimp with roasted bell peppers and onions

Description of the meal: Grilled shrimp with roasted bell peppers and onions is a delightful and colorful dish that highlights the natural flavors of shrimp and vegetables. The shrimp is marinated and grilled to perfection, while the bell peppers and onions are roasted to bring out their sweetness. This meal offers a balance of protein, vitamins, and minerals, making it a healthy and delicious option.

Ingredients:

- 1 pound large shrimp, peeled and deveined

- 2 tablespoons olive oil
- 2 cloves garlic, minced
- 1 teaspoon paprika
- 1/2 teaspoon cayenne pepper (optional, for heat)
- Salt and pepper to taste
- 2 bell peppers (assorted colors), sliced
- 1 large onion, sliced
- 1 tablespoon balsamic vinegar
- Fresh parsley, chopped (for garnish)

Instructions:

1. In a bowl, combine the olive oil, minced garlic, paprika, cayenne pepper (if using), salt, and pepper. Add the shrimp to the bowl and toss to coat. Let it marinate for about 15 minutes.

2. Preheat the grill to medium-high heat.

3. Thread the marinated shrimp onto skewers, evenly distributing them.

4. In a separate bowl, combine the sliced bell peppers and onions. Drizzle them with olive oil, balsamic vinegar, salt, and pepper. Toss to coat.

5. Place the bell peppers and onions on a grilling pan or aluminum foil.

6. Grill the shrimp skewers and the bell peppers and onions on the preheated grill. Cook the shrimp for about 2-3 minutes per side until they are opaque and cooked through. Grill the bell peppers and onions for about 6-8 minutes until they are tender and slightly charred.

7. Remove the shrimp skewers and grilled

vegetables from the grill.

8. Serve the grilled shrimp with roasted bell peppers and onions, garnished with fresh parsley.

Nutritional Information:

- Calories: 200
- Protein: 25g
- Fat: 8g
- Carbohydrates: 10g
- Fiber: 3g

Lemon herb roasted chicken breast with steamed asparagus

Description of the meal: Lemon herb roasted chicken breast with steamed asparagus is a flavorful and wholesome dish that combines juicy chicken breast with tender asparagus. The chicken breast is marinated in a tangy lemon herb mixture and then roasted to perfection. Served with steamed asparagus, this meal provides a satisfying balance of protein and vegetables.

Ingredients:

- 4 chicken breasts
- 2 tablespoons olive oil
- Juice of 1 lemon
- Zest of 1 lemon
- 2 cloves garlic, minced
- 1 teaspoon dried thyme
- 1 teaspoon dried rosemary
- Salt and pepper to taste
- 1 bunch asparagus, ends trimmed

- Lemon wedges (for serving)

Instructions:

1. Preheat the oven to 425°F (220°C).

2. In a bowl, whisk together the olive oil, lemon juice, lemon zest, minced garlic, dried thyme, dried rosemary, salt, and pepper.

3. Place the chicken breasts in a shallow dish and pour the marinade over them. Ensure the chicken breasts are coated evenly. Let them marinate for about 20-30 minutes.

4. Transfer the marinated chicken breasts to a baking dish lined with parchment paper.

5. Roast the chicken breasts in the preheated oven for about 25-30 minutes, or until they reach an internal temperature of 165°F (74°C) and the juices run clear. Flip the chicken breasts halfway through cooking.

6. While the chicken is roasting, steam the asparagus until it is tender-crisp, about 4-5 minutes.

7. Season the steamed asparagus with salt and pepper to taste.

8. Remove the chicken breasts from the oven and let them rest for a few minutes.

9. Serve the lemon herb roasted chicken breast with steamed asparagus.

10. Garnish with lemon wedges for added zest, if desired.

Nutritional Information:

- Calories: 300
- Protein: 40g
- Fat: 10g
- Carbohydrates: 5g
- Fiber: 3g

Baked halibut with garlic and herbs, accompanied by sautéed mushrooms

Description of the meal: Baked halibut with garlic and herbs is a flavorful and healthy dish that showcases the delicate flavor of halibut. The fish is seasoned with garlic and a blend of aromatic herbs, then baked to perfection. Served alongside sautéed mushrooms, this meal provides a delicious combination of protein and earthy flavors.

Ingredients:

- 4 halibut fillets
- Salt and pepper to taste
- 2 tablespoons olive oil
- 4 cloves garlic, minced
- 1 teaspoon dried thyme
- 1 teaspoon dried oregano
- 1/2 teaspoon paprika
- 1/2 teaspoon onion powder
- 1/4 teaspoon red pepper flakes (optional, for heat)
- 8 ounces mushrooms, sliced
- 2 tablespoons butter
- Fresh parsley, chopped (for garnish)

Instructions:

1. Preheat the oven to 400°F (200°C).

2. Season the halibut fillets with salt and pepper on both sides.

3. In a small bowl, combine the olive oil, minced garlic, dried thyme, dried oregano, paprika, onion powder, and red pepper flakes (if using).

4. Brush the halibut fillets with the garlic and herb mixture, coating them evenly.

5. Place the seasoned halibut fillets on a baking sheet lined with parchment paper.

6. Bake the halibut in the preheated oven for about 12-15 minutes, or until it is opaque and flakes easily with a fork.

7. While the halibut is baking, heat a skillet over medium-high heat.

8. Add the sliced mushrooms to the skillet and sauté for about 5-7 minutes, or until they are tender and golden brown.

9. Add the butter to the skillet and let it melt, coating the mushrooms.

10. Season the sautéed mushrooms with salt and pepper to taste.

11. Remove the halibut from the oven and let it rest for a few minutes.

12. Serve the baked halibut with garlic and herbs, accompanied by sautéed mushrooms.

13. Garnish with freshly chopped parsley.

Nutritional Information:

- Calories: 250
- Protein: 30g

- Fat: 12g
- Carbohydrates: 5g
- Fiber: 2g

Lean ground beef lettuce wraps with cucumber and tomato salad

Description of the meal: Lean ground beef lettuce wraps with cucumber and tomato salad is a light and refreshing meal that combines the savory flavors of seasoned ground beef with a crisp and tangy salad. The lettuce acts as a fresh and crunchy wrap, while the cucumber and tomato salad adds a burst of freshness. This meal is not only delicious but also provides a good balance of protein and vegetables.

Ingredients: For the lettuce wraps:

- 1 pound lean ground beef
- 1 tablespoon olive oil
- 1 onion, finely chopped
- 2 cloves garlic, minced
- 1 teaspoon ground cumin
- 1 teaspoon paprika
- 1/2 teaspoon chili powder (optional, for heat)
- Salt and pepper to taste
- Iceberg lettuce leaves

For the cucumber and tomato salad:

- 1 English cucumber, diced
- 2 tomatoes, diced

- 1/4 cup red onion, finely chopped
- 2 tablespoons fresh lemon juice
- 1 tablespoon olive oil
- 1 tablespoon chopped fresh parsley
- Salt and pepper to taste

Instructions: For the lettuce wraps:

1. Heat the olive oil in a large skillet over medium-high heat.

2. Add the chopped onion to the skillet and sauté until it becomes translucent.

3. Add the minced garlic to the skillet and cook for an additional 1-2 minutes until fragrant.

4. Add the lean ground beef to the skillet and cook, breaking it up with a spoon, until it is browned and cooked through.

5. Stir in the ground cumin, paprika, chili powder (if using), salt, and pepper. Cook for another 1-2 minutes to allow the flavors to meld.

6. Remove the skillet from the heat.

7. Prepare the lettuce leaves by carefully separating them, rinsing them, and patting them dry.

8. Spoon the cooked ground beef mixture onto each lettuce leaf.

9. Serve the lettuce wraps immediately.

For the cucumber and tomato salad:

1. In a bowl, combine the diced cucumber, diced tomatoes, finely chopped red onion, fresh lemon juice, olive oil, chopped fresh parsley, salt, and

pepper.

2. Toss the ingredients together until well combined.

3. Let the salad sit for a few minutes to allow the flavors to develop.

4. Serve the cucumber and tomato salad alongside the lettuce wraps.

Nutritional Information (per serving of lettuce wraps):

- Calories: 200
- Protein: 20g
- Fat: 10g
- Carbohydrates: 6g
- Fiber: 1g

Nutritional Information (per serving of cucumber and tomato salad):

- Calories: 40
- Protein: 1g
- Fat: 3g
- Carbohydrates: 4g
- Fiber: 1g

Grilled tuna steak with a side of sautéed kale

Description of the meal: Grilled tuna steak with a side of sautéed kale is a delicious and nutritious dish that highlights the natural flavors of the tuna and the earthy taste of kale. The tuna steak is marinated and grilled to perfection, resulting in a tender and flavorful centerpiece. Served with sautéed kale, this meal offers a balance of protein, vitamins, and minerals.

Ingredients:

- 2 tuna steaks
- 2 tablespoons soy sauce
- 1 tablespoon lemon juice
- 1 tablespoon olive oil
- 2 cloves garlic, minced
- 1/2 teaspoon black pepper
- Salt to taste
- 1 bunch kale, stems removed and leaves chopped
- 2 tablespoons olive oil
- 2 cloves garlic, minced
- Salt and pepper to taste
- Lemon wedges (for serving)

Instructions: For the grilled tuna steak:

1. In a shallow dish, combine the soy sauce, lemon juice, olive oil, minced garlic, black pepper, and salt.

2. Place the tuna steaks in the marinade and let them marinate for about 20 minutes, turning them once or twice to coat both sides.

3. Preheat the grill to medium-high heat.

4. Remove the tuna steaks from the marinade and discard the excess marinade.

5. Place the tuna steaks on the grill and cook for about 2-3 minutes per side for medium-rare, or adjust the cooking time to your desired doneness.

6. Remove the tuna steaks from the grill and let them rest for a few minutes.

7. Slice the tuna steaks into thick slices.

8. Serve the grilled tuna steak with lemon wedges on the side.

For the sautéed kale:

1. Heat the olive oil in a large skillet over medium heat.

2. Add the minced garlic to the skillet and sauté for about 1 minute until fragrant.

3. Add the chopped kale leaves to the skillet and cook, stirring occasionally, until the kale is wilted and tender, about 5-7 minutes.

4. Season the sautéed kale with salt and pepper to taste.

5. Remove the skillet from the heat.

6. Serve the sautéed kale alongside the grilled tuna steak.

Nutritional Information (per serving of grilled tuna steak):

- Calories: 250
- Protein: 30g
- Fat: 10g
- Carbohydrates: 2g
- Fiber: 0g

Nutritional Information (per serving of sautéed kale):

- Calories: 100
- Protein: 4g

- Fat: 7g
- Carbohydrates: 8g
- Fiber: 2g

Baked chicken drumsticks with roasted cauliflower

Description of the meal: Baked chicken drumsticks with roasted cauliflower is a hearty and satisfying dish that combines juicy chicken drumsticks with flavorful roasted cauliflower. The chicken drumsticks are seasoned with a blend of herbs and spices, then baked to perfection. Served alongside roasted cauliflower, this meal provides a delicious combination of protein and vegetables.

Ingredients:

- 8 chicken drumsticks
- 2 tablespoons olive oil
- 1 teaspoon garlic powder
- 1 teaspoon paprika
- 1/2 teaspoon dried thyme
- 1/2 teaspoon dried rosemary
- Salt and pepper to taste
- 1 head cauliflower, cut into florets
- 2 tablespoons olive oil
- 1 teaspoon cumin
- 1/2 teaspoon chili powder (optional, for heat)
- Salt and pepper to taste
- Fresh parsley, chopped (for garnish)

Instructions: For the baked chicken drumsticks:

1. Preheat the oven to 425°F (220°C).
2. In a small bowl, combine the olive oil, garlic

powder, paprika, dried thyme, dried rosemary, salt, and pepper to make a marinade.

3. Place the chicken drumsticks in a baking dish and pour the marinade over them. Ensure the drumsticks are coated evenly.

4. Bake the chicken drumsticks in the preheated oven for about 35-40 minutes, or until they are cooked through and the skin is golden brown.

5. Remove the chicken drumsticks from the oven and let them rest for a few minutes.

6. Serve the baked chicken drumsticks.

For the roasted cauliflower:

1. Preheat the oven to 425°F (220°C).

2. In a large bowl, toss the cauliflower florets with olive oil, cumin, chili powder (if using), salt, and pepper.

3. Spread the seasoned cauliflower florets in a single layer on a baking sheet.

4. Roast the cauliflower in the preheated oven for about 25-30 minutes, or until it is tender and lightly browned, stirring once halfway through.

5. Remove the roasted cauliflower from the oven.

6. Serve the roasted cauliflower alongside the baked chicken drumsticks.

7. Garnish with freshly chopped parsley.

Nutritional Information (per serving of baked chicken drumsticks):

- Calories: 250
- Protein: 30g
- Fat: 15g
- Carbohydrates: 1g
- Fiber: 0g

Nutritional Information (per serving of roasted cauliflower):

- Calories: 100
- Protein: 3g
- Fat: 7g
- Carbohydrates: 9g
- Fiber: 4g

Egg white omelette filled with mushrooms, spinach, and tomatoes

Description of the meal: An egg white omelette filled with mushrooms, spinach, and tomatoes is a nutritious and satisfying breakfast option. This omelette is made with egg whites, which are low in fat and cholesterol while being high in protein. The filling of mushrooms, spinach, and tomatoes adds a burst of flavor and a variety of vitamins and minerals. This meal is perfect for those looking for a healthy and delicious way to start their day.

Ingredients:

- 6 egg whites
- Salt and pepper to taste
- 1 tablespoon olive oil
- 1 cup sliced mushrooms
- 1 cup baby spinach leaves
- 1/2 cup cherry tomatoes, halved

- 2 tablespoons grated Parmesan cheese (optional)
- Fresh parsley, chopped (for garnish)

Instructions:

1. In a bowl, whisk the egg whites until frothy. Season with salt and pepper to taste.

2. Heat the olive oil in a non-stick skillet over medium heat.

3. Add the sliced mushrooms to the skillet and sauté for about 3-4 minutes, or until they are tender and lightly browned.

4. Add the baby spinach leaves to the skillet and cook until they are wilted.

5. Add the halved cherry tomatoes to the skillet and cook for another minute, just until they are heated through.

6. Remove the vegetables from the skillet and set them aside.

7. Reduce the heat to low and wipe the skillet clean.

8. Coat the skillet with cooking spray or a little extra olive oil.

9. Pour the whisked egg whites into the skillet and cook for about 2-3 minutes, or until the edges are set.

10. Carefully flip the omelette and cook for another 2-3 minutes, or until it is cooked through.

11. Transfer the omelette to a plate.

12. Spoon the sautéed mushrooms, spinach, and tomatoes onto one half of the omelette.

13. Sprinkle with grated Parmesan cheese if desired.

14. Fold the other half of the omelette over the filling to create a half-moon shape.

15. Garnish with freshly chopped parsley.

16. Serve the egg white omelette hot.

Nutritional Information:

- Calories: 150
- Protein: 20g
- Fat: 5g
- Carbohydrates: 5g
- Fiber: 2g

Grilled lean beef skewers with grilled zucchini and bell peppers

Description of the meal: Grilled lean beef skewers with grilled zucchini and bell peppers is a delicious and satisfying meal that brings together tender and flavorful beef with charred vegetables. The beef skewers are marinated in a savory blend of herbs and spices, then grilled to perfection. Paired with grilled zucchini and bell peppers, this meal offers a balance of protein and vibrant vegetables.

Ingredients: For the beef skewers:

- 1 pound lean beef, cut into cubes
- 2 tablespoons olive oil
- 2 cloves garlic, minced
- 1 teaspoon dried oregano
- 1 teaspoon paprika
- 1/2 teaspoon cumin

- Salt and pepper to taste
- Wooden skewers, soaked in water for 30 minutes

For the grilled zucchini and bell peppers:

- 2 zucchinis, sliced into thick rounds
- 2 bell peppers (any color), cut into chunks
- 2 tablespoons olive oil
- Salt and pepper to taste

Instructions: For the beef skewers:

1. In a bowl, combine the olive oil, minced garlic, dried oregano, paprika, cumin, salt, and pepper to make a marinade.

2. Add the beef cubes to the marinade and toss to coat them evenly. Let the beef marinate for at least 30 minutes, or overnight for more flavor.

3. Preheat the grill to medium-high heat.

4. Thread the marinated beef cubes onto the soaked wooden skewers.

5. Grill the beef skewers for about 8-10 minutes, turning them occasionally, until they are cooked to your desired level of doneness.

6. Remove the beef skewers from the grill and let them rest for a few minutes.

7. Serve the grilled beef skewers.

For the grilled zucchini and bell peppers:

1. Preheat the grill to medium-high heat.

2. In a bowl, toss the zucchini rounds and bell pepper chunks with olive oil, salt, and pepper.

3. Place the vegetables on the grill and cook for about

4-5 minutes per side, or until they are tender and have nice grill marks.

4. Remove the grilled zucchini and bell peppers from the grill.

5. Serve the grilled zucchini and bell peppers alongside the beef skewers.

Nutritional Information (per serving):

- Calories: 250
- Protein: 25g
- Fat: 12g
- Carbohydrates: 10g
- Fiber: 3g

Baked turkey breast with steamed snap peas

Description of the meal: Baked turkey breast with steamed snap peas is a nutritious and flavorful dish that showcases tender and juicy turkey breast alongside vibrant and crisp snap peas. The turkey breast is seasoned with herbs and spices, then baked to perfection. Served with steamed snap peas, this meal provides a balanced combination of protein and vegetables.

Ingredients:

- 1 pound turkey breast
- 1 tablespoon olive oil
- 1 teaspoon dried thyme
- 1 teaspoon dried rosemary
- 1/2 teaspoon garlic powder
- 1/2 teaspoon paprika
- Salt and pepper to taste

- 1 pound snap peas, trimmed
- 2 tablespoons water
- Salt and pepper to taste

Instructions: For the baked turkey breast:

1. Preheat the oven to 375°F (190°C).

2. Rub the turkey breast with olive oil, ensuring it is coated evenly.

3. In a small bowl, combine the dried thyme, dried rosemary, garlic powder, paprika, salt, and pepper.

4. Sprinkle the herb and spice mixture over the turkey breast, pressing it gently to adhere.

5. Place the seasoned turkey breast on a baking dish or roasting pan.

6. Bake the turkey breast in the preheated oven for about 45-55 minutes, or until it reaches an internal temperature of 165°F (74°C).

7. Remove the turkey breast from the oven and let it rest for a few minutes before slicing.

8. Slice the turkey breast into thick slices.

9. Serve the baked turkey breast.

For the steamed snap peas:

1. Place a steamer basket or colander over a pot filled with about an inch of water.

2. Bring the water to a boil.

3. Add the snap peas to the steamer basket or colander.

4. Cover the pot and steam the snap peas for about 2-3 minutes, or until they are crisp-tender.

5. Remove the steamed snap peas from the heat.

6. Season with salt and pepper to taste.

7. Serve the steamed snap peas alongside the baked turkey breast.

Nutritional Information (per serving of baked turkey breast):

- Calories: 200
- Protein: 40g
- Fat: 3g
- Carbohydrates: 0g
- Fiber: 0g

Nutritional Information (per serving of steamed snap peas):

- Calories: 50
- Protein: 2g
- Fat: 0g
- Carbohydrates: 10g
- Fiber: 4g

CHAPTER FOUR

*Understanding the
Role of Exercise*

Importance Of Physical Activity During The Scarsdale Diet

Physical activity plays a vital role in achieving optimal health and overall well-being. When combined with a healthy diet, it can significantly enhance the effectiveness of weight loss and contribute to maintaining a healthy weight in the long term. The Scarsdale Diet, known for its low-carbohydrate and high-protein approach, can benefit from incorporating regular physical activity. Let's explore the importance of physical activity during the Scarsdale Diet and how it can enhance your weight loss journey.

Regular exercise offers numerous benefits beyond weight loss. It improves cardiovascular health, boosts mood, increases energy levels, and helps prevent chronic diseases. When following the Scarsdale Diet, incorporating physical activity can further enhance these benefits and improve the overall outcome of the diet plan.

1. Enhances calorie burn: Physical activity increases energy expenditure, allowing you to burn more calories.

The Scarsdale Diet restricts calorie intake, and by adding exercise to the equation, you create a larger calorie deficit. This deficit is crucial for weight loss as it encourages your body to tap into stored fat for energy.

2. Preserves lean muscle mass: During weight loss, it is common to lose both fat and muscle. Regular exercise, particularly strength training, helps preserve lean muscle mass. This is important because muscle is metabolically active and helps increase your basal metabolic rate (BMR), leading to more efficient calorie burning even at rest.

3. Improves overall fitness: Physical activity during the Scarsdale Diet can improve your fitness levels, making everyday tasks easier and reducing the risk of injuries. Engaging in cardiovascular exercises such as brisk walking, jogging, or cycling can enhance your endurance, while strength training exercises like lifting weights or bodyweight exercises can improve your strength and muscle tone.

4. Supports mental well-being: Exercise has a positive impact on mental health and can help reduce stress, anxiety, and symptoms of depression. Following a diet plan can sometimes be challenging, and regular physical activity can serve as an outlet for stress, boost your mood, and provide a sense of accomplishment.

5. Sustains long-term weight management: One of the primary goals of the Scarsdale Diet is to help individuals achieve their desired weight and maintain it over time. Incorporating physical activity into your daily routine during the diet helps establish healthy habits and supports long-term weight management. Regular exercise helps prevent weight regain by increasing your calorie expenditure and supporting your overall metabolic health.

To maximize the benefits of physical activity during the Scarsdale Diet, it's essential to choose the right types of exercises and create a well-rounded exercise routine that complements the diet plan. The following section will provide recommendations for types of exercises and tips for creating an exercise routine that aligns with the Scarsdale Diet.

Recommended Types Of Exercises For Maximum Results

When selecting exercises to complement the Scarsdale Diet, it's important to focus on activities that maximize calorie burn, promote overall fitness, and are enjoyable to sustain long-term adherence. Here are some recommended types of exercises that can help you achieve maximum results:

1. Cardiovascular exercises: Activities that elevate your heart rate and increase your breathing rate are excellent for burning calories and improving cardiovascular health. Brisk walking, jogging, swimming, cycling, dancing, and aerobic classes are great options. Aim for at least 150 minutes of moderate-intensity cardio exercises per week or 75 minutes of vigorous-intensity exercises.

2. High-intensity interval training (HIIT): HIIT involves short bursts of intense exercises followed by periods of rest or low-intensity recovery. This type of training is time-efficient and can maximize calorie burn both during and after the workout. HIIT exercises can include sprint intervals, bodyweight circuits, or using equipment like kettlebells or dumbbells. Aim for 20-30 minutes of HIIT workouts, 2-3 times per week, to effectively enhance fat burning and improve cardiovascular fitness.

3. Strength training: Including strength training exercises in your routine helps build lean muscle mass, improve strength, and boost metabolism. Focus on compound exercises that work multiple muscle groups, such as squats, lunges, deadlifts, push-ups, and overhead presses. Aim for 2-3 strength training sessions per week, allowing a day of rest between sessions to allow muscles to recover and grow.

4. Flexibility and stretching: Don't forget to incorporate flexibility exercises into your routine to improve range of motion, prevent injuries, and promote relaxation. Activities such as yoga, Pilates, or static stretching can help improve flexibility and promote overall well-being. Consider adding a dedicated flexibility session to your weekly routine or incorporating stretching exercises after each workout.

5. Active lifestyle: In addition to structured exercise sessions, it's essential to maintain an active lifestyle throughout the day. Look for opportunities to be physically active in your daily routine, such as taking the stairs instead of the elevator, parking farther away from your destination, or going for a walk during your lunch break. These small lifestyle changes can add up and contribute to your overall physical activity level.

Creating An Exercise Routine That Complements The Diet

To create an exercise routine that complements the Scarsdale Diet, it's important to consider your fitness level, preferences, and availability. Here are some tips to help you design an exercise routine that aligns with the diet plan:

1. Set realistic goals: Determine what you want to achieve through your exercise routine, whether it's weight loss, improved fitness, or increased strength. Set specific and achievable goals to keep yourself motivated and track your progress.

2. Consult a professional: If you're new to exercise or have any underlying health conditions, it's advisable to consult a healthcare professional or a certified fitness trainer. They can provide personalized guidance, tailor exercises to your needs, and ensure you perform them safely and effectively.

3. Balance cardio and strength training: Include a combination of cardiovascular exercises and strength training in your routine to optimize results. Cardio exercises burn calories and improve cardiovascular health, while strength training helps build lean muscle mass and increase metabolism. Aim for a balanced approach that incorporates both types of exercises.

4. Plan your workouts: Schedule your workouts in advance to ensure consistency. Decide on the days and times that work best for you and treat them as non-negotiable appointments with yourself. Having a structured plan increases the likelihood of sticking to your exercise routine.

5. Gradually increase intensity: Start at a comfortable intensity and gradually increase the intensity and duration of your workouts over time. This progressive approach helps prevent injuries and allows your body to adapt to the new demands.

6. Find activities you enjoy: Choose exercises that you genuinely enjoy to make your routine more sustainable and enjoyable. Whether it's dancing, swimming, hiking, or playing a sport, find activities that keep you motivated and excited to stay active.

Tips For Staying Motivated And Maintaining An Active Lifestyle

Motivation is key to maintaining an active lifestyle alongside the Scarsdale Diet. Here are some tips to help you stay motivated and make physical activity a consistent part of your daily routine:

1. Set short-term and long-term goals: Set both short-term and long-term goals related to your physical activity. Short-term goals can be weekly or monthly targets, such as increasing the duration of your workout or trying a new exercise. Long-term goals can be related to weight loss, strength gains, or completing a specific fitness event. Having goals to work towards provides a sense of purpose and motivation.

2. Track your progress: Keep track of your workouts, measurements, and achievements. Seeing your progress over time can be incredibly motivating and help you stay on track. Use a workout journal, a fitness app, or simply a calendar to record your activities and monitor your improvements.

3. Find an accountability partner: Consider partnering up with a friend or family member who shares similar fitness goals. Having someone to exercise with or share your progress with can provide mutual support and accountability. You can also join fitness classes or online communities to connect with like-minded individuals.

4. Mix it up: Avoid monotony by regularly changing your

exercise routine. Try new activities, vary your workouts, and explore different fitness classes or outdoor exercises. This helps prevent boredom and keeps you engaged and motivated.

5. Reward yourself: Celebrate your achievements and milestones along the way. Treat yourself to a non-food reward for reaching your goals, such as buying new workout gear, booking a massage, or enjoying a relaxing day at the spa. Rewards reinforce positive behavior and can help you stay motivated.

6. Make it enjoyable: Find ways to make your workouts enjoyable and fun. Listen to energizing music, podcasts, or audiobooks during your workouts. Create a workout playlist with your favorite songs that motivate you. Consider incorporating activities you enjoy, such as dancing, playing a sport, or exploring nature while hiking or cycling.

7. Schedule active breaks: Incorporate short bursts of physical activity throughout your day, especially if you have a sedentary job. Take regular breaks to stretch, walk around, or do a quick bodyweight exercise routine. These active breaks not only help burn extra calories but also energize your body and mind.

8. Stay flexible: Life can sometimes get in the way of your planned workouts. Be flexible and adaptable to changes in your schedule. If you miss a workout, don't dwell on it but focus on getting back on track as soon as possible.

9. Listen to your body: Pay attention to your body's needs and signals. Rest when you feel fatigued or sore. Push yourself, but also respect your limits to avoid injuries. Remember that a consistent and sustainable approach to exercise is more important than pushing yourself to the point of exhaustion.

10. Celebrate non-scale victories: Acknowledge and celebrate the non-scale victories that come with an active lifestyle, such as increased energy levels, improved sleep, reduced stress, or enhanced overall well-being. These positive changes are equally important as weight loss and can serve as powerful motivators.

By recognizing the importance of physical activity during the Scarsdale Diet, incorporating recommended types of exercises, creating a well-rounded exercise routine, and staying motivated, you can maximize your results and enjoy the benefits of an active lifestyle. Remember to consult with a healthcare professional before starting any new exercise program, especially if you have any pre-existing health conditions.

In addition to the tips mentioned earlier, here are a few more strategies to help you stay motivated and maintain an active lifestyle during the Scarsdale Diet:

1. Set reminders and create a schedule: Use reminders on your phone or set alarms to remind yourself of your scheduled workouts. Treat them as important appointments that you cannot miss. Having a consistent schedule can help establish a routine and make physical activity a regular part of your day.

2. Find a workout buddy: Exercising with a friend or family member can make your workouts more enjoyable and provide an extra layer of motivation. You can encourage and support each other, push each other to reach new goals, and make your exercise sessions more social.

3. Track your steps: Consider using a pedometer or a

fitness tracker to monitor your daily steps. Setting a goal to achieve a certain number of steps each day can motivate you to incorporate more physical activity into your routine. Take the stairs instead of the elevator, go for short walks during breaks, or park farther away from your destination to increase your step count.

4. Join fitness challenges or programs: Participating in fitness challenges or signing up for exercise programs can provide structure, accountability, and a sense of community. Look for local fitness events, virtual challenges, or online fitness programs that align with your goals and interests. These can help keep you motivated and engaged as you work towards achieving your desired results.

5. Mix up your workouts: Incorporating variety into your exercise routine can prevent boredom and keep you motivated. Explore different types of exercises, try new fitness classes, or switch up your workout locations. You can also alternate between indoor and outdoor activities to add excitement and keep things fresh.

6. Set rewards for achieving milestones: Set small rewards for yourself as you achieve various milestones along your fitness journey. For example, treat yourself to a new workout outfit, a massage, a day at the spa, or a fun activity you enjoy. Having something to look forward to can provide extra motivation to stay consistent with your exercise routine.

7. Use technology to your advantage: Take advantage of the numerous fitness apps, online workout videos, and digital resources available today. These tools can provide you with workout ideas, track your progress, offer guided workouts, and even connect you with virtual fitness communities. Find the ones that resonate with you and integrate them into your routine.

8. Practice self-care: Taking care of yourself goes beyond just physical activity. Make sure you prioritize self-care activities such as getting enough sleep, managing stress, and maintaining a balanced lifestyle. When you feel your best mentally and emotionally, it becomes easier to stay motivated and maintain an active lifestyle.

Remember, staying motivated and maintaining an active lifestyle is a journey, and there may be times when you face challenges or setbacks. During those times, remind yourself of the reasons why you started and the benefits you have experienced so far. Be patient with yourself, celebrate your progress, and stay focused on your long-term health and well-being.

By recognizing the importance of physical activity during the Scarsdale Diet and implementing strategies to stay motivated, you can create a healthy and sustainable lifestyle that supports your weight loss and overall health goals.

CHAPTER FIVE

*Addressing Common
Challenges and Concerns*

Dealing With Hunger And Food Cravings

Hunger and food cravings are common challenges that individuals face when trying to maintain a healthy diet or lose weight. Understanding how to effectively deal with these cravings is essential for long-term success. Here are some strategies to help manage hunger and food cravings:

1. Eat balanced meals: One of the most effective ways to prevent hunger and cravings is to eat balanced meals that include a combination of protein, healthy fats, and fiber-rich carbohydrates. These nutrients provide satiety and help stabilize blood sugar levels, reducing the likelihood of sudden cravings.

2. Stay hydrated: Sometimes, feelings of hunger can be mistaken for thirst. Ensure you drink enough water throughout the day to stay hydrated. Drinking water before meals can also help you feel fuller and reduce the chances of overeating.

3. Include protein in your meals: Protein is known to be more filling than carbohydrates or fats. Including adequate amounts of protein in your meals can help curb hunger and keep you satisfied for longer. Good sources of protein include lean meats, poultry, fish, tofu, legumes, and dairy products.

4. Choose high-fiber foods: Foods high in fiber take longer to digest, promoting a feeling of fullness and reducing hunger. Incorporate fruits, vegetables, whole grains, and legumes into your diet to increase fiber intake.

5. Practice mindful eating: Paying attention to your food and eating mindfully can help you recognize true hunger and distinguish it from emotional or boredom-driven cravings. Slow down, savor each bite, and listen to your body's cues of satiety.

6. Plan and prepare meals in advance: Planning and preparing meals in advance can help you make healthier choices and reduce impulsive food cravings. Having nutritious options readily available can prevent you from reaching for unhealthy snacks or takeout.

7. Use portion control: Monitoring portion sizes is crucial for managing hunger and cravings. Eating smaller, balanced portions can help you satisfy your hunger without consuming excessive calories. Use smaller plates or bowls to create an illusion of a fuller plate.

8. Identify trigger foods: Certain foods may trigger intense cravings or overeating. Identify these trigger foods and find healthier alternatives or strategies to manage your cravings when faced with them. For example, if you crave sweets, opt for a piece of dark chocolate or a naturally sweet fruit.

9. Practice stress management: Stress and emotions can often lead to unhealthy eating habits and cravings. Explore stress management techniques such as exercise, meditation, deep breathing, or engaging in activities you enjoy to help alleviate stress and reduce emotional eating.

10. Seek support: Surround yourself with a supportive network of friends, family, or a community who share similar goals. Sharing experiences, challenges, and strategies can provide valuable insights and help you stay motivated on your journey to managing hunger and cravings.

Remember, it's important to approach hunger and food cravings with a balanced mindset. Completely depriving yourself or labeling certain foods as "bad" can create an unhealthy relationship with food. Instead, focus on nourishing your body with wholesome foods while allowing occasional indulgences in moderation.

Overcoming Plateaus And Maintaining Weight Loss

Hitting a weight loss plateau can be frustrating and demotivating, but it's a common occurrence on any weight loss journey. However, with the right approach, you can overcome plateaus and continue progressing towards your weight loss goals. Here are some strategies to help you break through plateaus and maintain weight loss:

1. Evaluate your calorie intake: As you lose weight, your body's calorie needs may decrease. Reassess your calorie intake and make adjustments if necessary. Consider consulting a registered dietitian who can help you create a personalized plan based on your specific needs and goals.

2. Vary your exercise routine: When it comes to overcoming plateaus, changing up your exercise routine can make a significant difference. Your body can adapt to repetitive movements, leading to fewer calories burned. Incorporate different types of exercises, such as strength training, cardiovascular exercises, and HIIT (High-Intensity Interval Training), to challenge your body and boost your metabolism.

3. Increase intensity or duration: If you've been following the same exercise routine for a while, it might be time to increase the intensity or duration of your workouts. Push yourself a little harder by lifting heavier weights, increasing the speed or resistance on cardio machines, or extending the duration of your exercise sessions. This change can help break through the plateau and stimulate further weight loss.

4. Monitor your portion sizes: It's essential to maintain portion control even after reaching a plateau. Gradually reducing portion sizes or tracking your food intake using a food diary or mobile app can help you stay mindful of your calorie consumption and prevent overeating.

5. Focus on strength training: Incorporating strength training into your exercise routine can be particularly beneficial during plateaus. Building muscle mass increases your metabolism and helps you burn more calories even at rest. Include exercises that target major muscle groups, such as squats, lunges, deadlifts, and push-ups.

6. Prioritize sleep and stress management: Adequate sleep and stress management are often overlooked but critical factors in weight loss. Lack of sleep can affect hunger hormones, leading to increased cravings and a slower metabolism. Aim for 7-9 hours of quality sleep each night and find stress management techniques that work for you, such as meditation, yoga, or engaging in hobbies you enjoy.

7. Track your progress: Keep track of your measurements, body weight, and body composition to monitor your progress accurately. Sometimes, the scale may not budge, but your body composition may be changing positively. By focusing on overall health improvements rather than just the number on the scale, you can stay motivated and committed to your weight loss journey.

Handling Social Situations and Dining Out

Social situations and dining out can present challenges when you're trying to stick to a healthy eating plan. However, with some strategies and mindful choices, you can navigate these situations while still enjoying social interactions. Here are some tips for handling social situations and dining out:

1. Plan ahead: If you know you'll be attending a social event or dining out, plan ahead by checking the menu in advance. Look for healthier options and decide what you'll order before you arrive. Having a plan in place can help you make better choices and avoid impulsive decisions.

2. Communicate your goals: Let your friends, family, or dining companions know about your health goals and dietary preferences. By communicating your intentions, they can be supportive and understanding, making it easier for you to stick to your plan.

3. Choose restaurants wisely: Opt for restaurants that offer healthier menu options or customizable dishes. Look for places that focus on fresh, whole foods and have lighter options available. Ethnic cuisines like Mediterranean or Asian often have healthier choices with plenty of vegetables, lean proteins, and flavorful spices.

4. Practice portion control: Restaurant portions tend to be larger than what we need, leading to overeating. Be mindful of portion sizes and consider sharing a meal with a friend or requesting a smaller portion. You can also ask for a to-go box at the beginning of the meal and pack up half of your plate to enjoy later.

5. Make special requests: Don't be afraid to make special requests when ordering. Ask for dressings or sauces on the side, opt for grilled or steamed preparations instead of fried, and request substitutions like steamed vegetables instead of fries. Most restaurants are accommodating and willing to meet your dietary needs.

6. Be mindful of liquid calories: Alcoholic beverages, sugary sodas, and fancy coffee drinks can add a significant number of calories. Choose water, unsweetened tea, or sparkling water with a splash of citrus as your main beverage. If you do choose to have alcohol, opt for lighter options like a glass of wine or a vodka soda with fresh lime.

7. Fill up on vegetables: Look for dishes that incorporate plenty of vegetables, either as a main course or as side dishes. Vegetables are low in calories, high in fiber, and packed with nutrients. They can help you feel satisfied while still enjoying a delicious meal.

8. Practice mindful eating: Pay attention to your hunger and fullness cues, and eat slowly. Engage in conversation and savor each bite. By being mindful and present, you're less likely to overeat or make impulsive choices.

9. Choose quality over quantity: Instead of focusing solely on quantity, prioritize the quality of the food you're consuming. Seek out nutrient-dense options that nourish your body, rather than empty calories that provide little nutritional value.

10. Be flexible and forgiving: Remember that one meal or social event won't make or break your progress. If you indulge a bit more than planned, forgive yourself and get back on track with your next meal or activity. It's important to have a healthy balance between enjoying social occasions and staying committed to your goals.

By implementing these strategies, you can navigate social situations and dining out while maintaining a healthy eating plan. Remember that it's about making mindful choices, enjoying the experience, and finding a balance that works for you.

CHAPTER SIX

Tracking Weight Loss And Body Measurements

Tracking weight loss and body measurements is a crucial aspect of any successful weight management journey. While the number on the scale may be the most commonly used metric to gauge progress, it's essential to recognize that weight loss is not solely determined by the scale. By incorporating body measurements into your tracking routine, you can gain a more comprehensive understanding of your body's transformation.

Body Measurements Offer Several Advantages In Weight Management:

1. **Comprehensive Progress Assessment:** Relying solely on weight can be misleading, as it doesn't account for changes in body composition. By measuring various body parts such as waist, hips, chest, arms, and thighs, you can identify changes

in specific areas and understand how your body is transforming.

2. **Motivation Boost:** Seeing progress in body measurements, even when the scale doesn't budge, can provide a significant motivational boost. It reminds you that you're making positive changes and can keep you motivated to continue your journey.

3. **Accuracy in Tracking:** Body measurements provide a more accurate reflection of your body's changes over time. While weight can fluctuate due to factors like water retention or muscle gain, measurements tend to be more consistent and reliable indicators of progress.

When tracking weight loss and body measurements, consistency is key. Here are some tips to ensure accurate and meaningful measurements:

- Use a flexible measuring tape: A flexible measuring tape allows you to measure different body parts accurately. It's important to measure each area at the same spot consistently to get reliable results.

- Measure under the same conditions: To ensure consistency, measure yourself at the same time of day, preferably in the morning before eating or drinking. This eliminates potential fluctuations caused by food or water intake.

- Take measurements at regular intervals: Set a schedule to measure yourself, such as once a month or every two weeks. This interval provides enough time to see significant changes while avoiding becoming fixated on day-to-day fluctuations.

Remember, tracking weight loss and body measurements should be viewed as a tool for self-improvement rather than an obsession. Focus on the overall trends and the way you feel in your body, as these factors matter more than any number on a scale or measuring tape. By combining weight and body measurements, you can better understand your progress and celebrate the positive changes happening within you.

Understanding The Significance Of Non-Scale Victories

In the journey of weight loss and overall well-being, it's essential to recognize and celebrate non-scale victories (NSVs). NSVs refer to the positive changes and achievements that occur as a result of adopting a healthier lifestyle, regardless of the number on the scale. These victories encompass a wide range of accomplishments, both physical and psychological, that contribute to your overall well-being. Understanding the significance of NSVs can significantly impact your mindset and motivation throughout your journey.

Here are some examples of non-scale victories:

1. **Increased Energy Levels:** One of the most common NSVs is experiencing higher energy levels and improved stamina. As you adopt healthier habits and become more physically active, you may notice an increase in energy throughout the day, allowing you to accomplish tasks more efficiently and enjoy an overall improved quality of life.

2. **Improved Sleep Quality:** Adopting healthier

habits, such as regular exercise and a balanced diet, can positively impact your sleep patterns. Better sleep quality leads to increased alertness, improved mood, and enhanced cognitive function, contributing to your overall well-being.

3. **Clothing Fit and Body Shape Changes:** NSVs are often evident in changes in the way your clothes fit and alterations in your body shape. You may notice that your clothes feel looser, or you might need to buy a smaller size. These changes indicate progress in your journey and can boost your confidence and self-esteem.

4. **Improved Physical Fitness:** NSVs can be seen in improved physical fitness and athletic performance. You may notice that you can walk, run, or exercise for longer periods without feeling fatigued. Achieving milestones like running a certain distance, lifting heavier weights, or completing a challenging workout can be significant NSVs that highlight your progress and dedication.

5. **Positive Changes in Body Composition:** While the scale may not show significant changes, NSVs can manifest as improvements in body composition. By adopting a healthier lifestyle, you may notice a decrease in body fat percentage and an increase in muscle mass. These changes can lead to a more toned and defined physique, even if the scale doesn't reflect significant weight loss.

6. **Better Emotional Well-being:** NSVs extend beyond physical changes and can have a profound impact on your emotional well-being. As you

make healthier choices, you may experience reduced stress levels, improved mood, and increased self-confidence. These positive shifts in your mental and emotional state contribute to your overall happiness and satisfaction with your weight loss journey.

Understanding the significance of non-scale victories is crucial for maintaining motivation and a positive mindset throughout your journey. While the number on the scale can fluctuate and may not always reflect your efforts accurately, NSVs provide tangible evidence of the positive changes happening within your body and mind. Celebrate and embrace these victories, no matter how small they may seem, as they are vital milestones on the path to a healthier and happier life.

Evaluating The Effectiveness Of The Scarsdale Diet

The Scarsdale Diet is a popular weight loss plan that gained attention in the 1970s. Developed by Dr. Herman Tarnower, the diet emphasizes high-protein, low-carbohydrate, and low-calorie meals. It claims to provide rapid weight loss while maintaining muscle mass and promoting a balanced nutrient intake. However, it's important to evaluate the effectiveness and potential drawbacks of any diet before embarking on it.

Key points to consider when evaluating the effectiveness of the Scarsdale Diet:

1. **Initial Weight Loss:** The Scarsdale Diet is known for its promise of rapid weight loss. The strict calorie restriction and low carbohydrate intake

can lead to a significant initial drop in weight. However, it's crucial to recognize that much of this initial weight loss is often due to water weight and glycogen depletion rather than actual fat loss.

2. **Short-term vs. Long-term Results:** While the Scarsdale Diet may yield quick results in the short term, its long-term effectiveness is questionable. The strict rules and limited food choices can make it challenging to sustain over an extended period. Many people find it difficult to adhere to such a restrictive plan, leading to weight regain once they return to their regular eating habits.

3. **Nutritional Imbalance:** The Scarsdale Diet focuses on high protein and low carbohydrate intake, which can result in a nutritional imbalance. By severely restricting certain food groups, you may miss out on essential nutrients like fiber, vitamins, and minerals. This imbalance can potentially lead to deficiencies and negatively impact your overall health.

4. **Lack of Individualization:** The Scarsdale Diet is a one-size-fits-all approach that doesn't consider individual differences in metabolism, preferences, and dietary needs. What works for one person may not work for another. Sustainable weight loss is best achieved through personalized approaches that take into account an individual's unique circumstances.

5. **Sustainability and Lifestyle Adaptation:** The Scarsdale Diet may be challenging to sustain in the long run, as it restricts many foods and limits

variety. Successful weight management requires a sustainable and adaptable approach that can be incorporated into your lifestyle without feeling deprived or restricted.

It's important to approach any diet, including the Scarsdale Diet, with caution and carefully consider its potential impact on your overall health and well-being. While the Scarsdale Diet may offer short-term weight loss benefits, it's crucial to assess its long-term sustainability and nutritional adequacy.

Alternatives to the Scarsdale Diet: Instead of following a highly restrictive and unbalanced diet like the Scarsdale Diet, consider adopting a more balanced and sustainable approach to eating. Here are some strategies to consider:

1. **Focus on Whole Foods:** Emphasize whole, unprocessed foods in your diet, including fruits, vegetables, lean proteins, whole grains, and healthy fats. These foods provide essential nutrients and promote long-term health.

2. **Mindful Eating:** Pay attention to your body's hunger and fullness cues. Eat when you're hungry and stop when you're comfortably satisfied. Mindful eating helps you develop a healthier relationship with food and promotes better portion control.

3. **Moderation and Portion Control:** Rather than completely eliminating certain foods, practice moderation and portion control. Allow yourself to enjoy your favorite treats occasionally while being mindful of portion sizes.

4. **Regular Physical Activity:** Incorporate regular

exercise into your routine to support overall health and weight management. Find activities you enjoy and make them a regular part of your lifestyle.

5. **Seek Professional Guidance:** If you're struggling with weight loss or have specific dietary needs, consider consulting a registered dietitian or nutritionist. They can provide personalized guidance and help you develop a sustainable eating plan that suits your individual needs and preferences.

Remember, sustainable weight loss is not about following a short-term fad diet but adopting long-term lifestyle changes. Focus on nourishing your body with nutritious foods, staying physically active, and nurturing a positive relationship with food. By embracing a balanced and sustainable approach to eating, you can achieve lasting weight management and overall well-being.

Strategies For Weight Maintenance And Preventing Relapse

Weight maintenance is a critical phase of any weight loss journey, as it involves sustaining the achieved results over the long term. However, maintaining weight loss can be challenging, and many individuals experience relapses or regain the weight they worked hard to lose. To prevent relapse and successfully maintain a healthy weight, it's important to implement effective strategies that support long-term weight management.

Here are some strategies for weight maintenance and preventing relapse:

1. **Establish Realistic Goals:** Set realistic and sustainable weight maintenance goals. Rather than striving for a specific number on the scale, focus on maintaining a healthy lifestyle and overall well-being. Setting unattainable or overly strict goals can lead to frustration and an increased risk of relapse.

2. **Consistency in Habits:** Maintain the healthy habits that helped you achieve weight loss in the first place. This includes regular physical activity, mindful eating, and balanced nutrition. Consistency is key to preventing weight regain.

3. **Monitor Your Weight:** Regularly monitor your weight to catch any small fluctuations early on. This can help you identify potential issues and take corrective actions promptly. However, remember that weight naturally fluctuates, and it's essential to look at overall trends rather than day-to-day variations.

4. **Stay Active:** Continue engaging in regular physical activity even after reaching your weight loss goal. Exercise not only supports weight maintenance but also provides numerous health benefits, including improved cardiovascular health, increased strength, and enhanced mood.

5. **Practice Mindful Eating:** Continue practicing mindful eating techniques to maintain a healthy relationship with food. Pay attention to your body's hunger and fullness cues, eat slowly, and savor your meals. Avoid mindless eating and emotional eating, which can contribute to weight regain.

6. **Build a Support System:** Surround yourself with a supportive network of friends, family, or a weight loss maintenance group. Having a support system can provide encouragement, accountability, and guidance during challenging times.

7. **Address Emotional Triggers:** Identify and address emotional triggers that may lead to overeating or unhealthy behaviors. Develop alternative coping strategies such as exercise, engaging in hobbies, practicing relaxation techniques, or seeking professional support if needed.

8. **Celebrate Non-Scale Victories:** Continue to recognize and celebrate non-scale victories throughout your weight maintenance journey. These can serve as powerful motivators and reinforce your healthy habits and progress.

9. **Regular Self-Reflection:** Engage in regular self-reflection to assess your mindset, habits, and progress. Identify any potential areas for improvement or areas where you may be slipping into old habits. Adjust your strategies as needed to maintain a healthy lifestyle.

10. **Plan for Challenges:** Anticipate and plan for potential challenges that may arise, such as vacations, holidays, or stressful periods. Prepare strategies in advance to navigate these situations while staying on track with your weight maintenance goals.

Remember, weight maintenance is a lifelong commitment, and it's natural to encounter ups and downs along the way.

Embrace a positive mindset, be kind to yourself, and view setbacks as learning opportunities rather than failures. By implementing these strategies and maintaining a healthy lifestyle, you can increase your chances of long-term weight maintenance and prevent relapse.

Embracing A Balanced And Sustainable Approach To Eating

When it comes to achieving and maintaining a healthy weight, it's essential to embrace a balanced and sustainable approach to eating. Fad diets and extreme restrictions may offer short-term results, but they are rarely sustainable or beneficial for long-term health. Instead, focusing on nourishing your body with a variety of nutrient-dense foods and adopting healthy eating habits can lead to lasting success.

Here are key principles to consider when embracing a balanced and sustainable approach to eating:

1. **Incorporate Nutrient-Dense Foods:** Prioritize nutrient-dense foods that provide a wide range of essential nutrients, including fruits, vegetables, whole grains, lean proteins, and healthy fats. These foods not only support weight management but also contribute to overall health and well-being.

2. **Practice Portion Control:** Pay attention to portion sizes and practice mindful eating. Be aware of your body's hunger and fullness cues to prevent overeating. It's helpful to use smaller plates and bowls and take your time to savor each bite.

3. **Include All Food Groups:** Avoid excluding entire food groups unless medically necessary. Each food group offers unique nutrients that are essential for a well-balanced diet. Aim for a variety of fruits, vegetables, whole grains, lean proteins, and low-fat dairy or dairy alternatives.

4. **Moderation, Not Deprivation:** Instead of completely depriving yourself of certain foods, practice moderation. Allow yourself to enjoy your favorite treats occasionally, but be mindful of portion sizes and frequency. This approach helps prevent feelings of deprivation and reduces the likelihood of binging or falling into unhealthy eating patterns.

5. **Mindful Eating:** Develop a mindful eating practice by paying attention to your eating experience. Slow down, savor the flavors, and listen to your body's hunger and fullness signals. By being present in the moment, you can better enjoy your meals and make conscious choices.

6. **Hydration:** Stay hydrated by drinking an adequate amount of water throughout the day. Water is essential for various bodily functions and can help manage appetite and cravings. Limit sugary beverages and opt for water as your primary source of hydration.

7. **Meal Planning and Preparation:** Plan and prepare meals in advance to support healthier choices. This practice can help you avoid relying on convenience or fast foods, which tend to be less nutritious. Consider batch cooking, meal prepping, or using meal delivery services to

simplify the process.

8. **Listen to Your Body:** Tune in to your body's signals of hunger, fullness, and satisfaction. Eat when you're hungry and stop when you're comfortably satisfied, avoiding overeating. Allow yourself to enjoy a wide variety of foods while being mindful of how they make you feel.

9. **Seek Professional Guidance:** If you're unsure about how to create a balanced and sustainable eating plan, consider consulting a registered dietitian or nutritionist. They can provide personalized recommendations based on your specific needs, preferences, and health goals.

10. **Lifestyle Approach:** Adopt a long-term lifestyle approach rather than viewing your eating habits as a temporary diet. Sustainable weight management and overall health require consistent healthy choices that can be incorporated into your everyday life.

By embracing a balanced and sustainable approach to eating, you can nourish your body, achieve your weight goals, and improve your overall well-being. Remember, healthy eating is a journey, and it's important to be patient and kind to yourself along the way.

CONCLUSION

Recap Of The Key Points Covered In The Ebook

In this ebook, we have explored the Scarsdale Diet and its potential benefits for individuals looking to lose weight and adopt a healthier lifestyle. Throughout the chapters, we have discussed various aspects of the diet, including its principles, recommended food choices, and the suggested meal plan. Let's recap the key points covered so far.

1. The Scarsdale Diet principles: The Scarsdale Diet is a high-protein, low-carbohydrate, and low-calorie diet designed to promote weight loss. It emphasizes the consumption of lean proteins, fruits, and vegetables while limiting the intake of carbohydrates and fats. By following this dietary approach, individuals can achieve rapid weight loss results.

2. Balanced meal plan: The Scarsdale Diet provides a balanced meal plan that includes a variety of foods from different food groups. The daily menu consists of lean proteins such as fish, poultry, and lean meats, as well as fruits and vegetables. The diet also incorporates a specific portion size for each food group to ensure a well-balanced intake of nutrients.

3. Limited calorie intake: One of the key aspects of the Scarsdale Diet is its restricted calorie intake. The diet typically allows for around 1,000 to 1,200 calories per day, which is considerably lower than the average daily caloric intake. By consuming fewer calories, the body is forced to use stored fat for energy, resulting in weight loss.

4. Emphasis on protein: The Scarsdale Diet places a strong emphasis on protein-rich foods. Protein is known to provide satiety, helping individuals feel fuller for longer periods. Moreover, protein plays a crucial role in building and repairing tissues, maintaining muscle mass, and supporting overall health.

5. Carbohydrate restriction: The Scarsdale Diet restricts the consumption of carbohydrates, especially refined carbohydrates and sugars. By reducing carbohydrate intake, the diet aims to control blood sugar levels and promote weight loss. Instead of relying on carbohydrates for energy, the body utilizes stored fat as a source of fuel.

6. Regular physical activity: While the Scarsdale Diet primarily focuses on dietary changes, incorporating regular physical activity is encouraged. Exercise not only aids in weight loss but also promotes overall health and well-being. Engaging in activities such as brisk walking, cycling, or strength training can complement the diet and enhance its effectiveness.

Encouragement And Motivation For Readers

Embarking on a new diet and lifestyle change can be challenging, but it's important to stay motivated and focused on your goals. Here are some words of encouragement and motivation to support you on your journey.

1. Set realistic goals: Remember that weight loss is a gradual process, and setting realistic goals is crucial. Rather than aiming for rapid, unsustainable weight loss, focus on making long-term, sustainable changes to your eating habits and lifestyle. Celebrate small milestones along the way to keep your motivation high.

2. Find a support system: Surround yourself with a supportive network of friends, family, or fellow dieters. Having a support system can provide encouragement, accountability, and a space to share your challenges and successes. Consider joining online communities or local groups where you can connect with individuals on a similar journey.

3. Stay positive: A positive mindset is essential when adopting any lifestyle change. Instead of focusing on what you can't eat or the challenges you may encounter, shift your focus to the benefits and positive outcomes you are working towards. Remind yourself of your motivations and the reasons why you chose to follow the Scarsdale Diet.

www.ingramcontent.com/pod-product-compliance
Lightning Source LLC
Chambersburg PA
CBHW050930260726
48660CB00001B/493